Ana Carla Silva dos Santos
José Carlos G. C. Leitão

Physical Exercise for the Elderly with Hypertension

Ana Carla Silva dos Santos
José Carlos G. C. Leitão

Physical Exercise for the Elderly with Hypertension

Cardiovascular Benefits

ScienciaScripts

Imprint

Cover image: www.ingimage.com

This book is a translation from the original published under ISBN 978-613-9-73298-2.

Publisher:
Sciencia Scripts
is a trademark of
Dodo Books Indian Ocean Ltd. and OmniScriptum S.R.L publishing group

120 High Road, East Finchley, London, N2 9ED, United Kingdom
Str. Armeneasca 28/1, office 1, Chisinau MD-2012, Republic of Moldova, Europe
Printed at: see last page
ISBN: 978-620-7-88865-8

Thank you

I thank God for his strength and discernment in the realisation of this achievement and I ask him for wisdom to achieve new conquests.

To my parents, Fátima Cabral and José Erinaldo, for their love and unconditional support, even in the most difficult times, always committed to my professional fulfilment, even if this required great sacrifices.

To my sister Flavyana Santos for also being part of this journey and for giving me a beautiful niece, Ana Flávya, who sometimes made me smile at the most tense moments.

I would like to thank my entire team at the Cardiological Emergency Department of Pernambuco - PROCAPE.

To José Carlos Gomes Leitão, PhD, for all his encouragement and dedication. There are few words to express the affection and admiration I have for this person.

CONTENTS

INTRODUCTION

According to the criteria of the World Health Organisation (WHO), the elderly are those aged at least 60 years or over, while in developing and developed countries the elderly are those aged 65 years or over.

Brazil is a country where the growth of the elderly population has outstripped population growth. Currently, the 80+ age group is made up of 2,935,585 people (IBGE, 2011), representing 14 per cent of Brazil's elderly population.

According to the Population Reference Bureau (2011), the countries with the most elderly people are Japan 23.2%, Germany 20.7%, Italy 20.2%, Greece 18.9%, Sweden 18.5%, Portugal 17.9%, Bulgaria 17.7%, Austria 17.6, Finland 17.5%, Latvia 17.4%. In Brazil, on the other hand, the representation of age groups in relation to the total population in 2010 is lower than that observed in 2000 for all age groups up to 25 years old, while the other age groups have increased their participation in the last decade. As a result, we can see that the relative share of the population aged 65 and over has grown from 4.8 per cent in 1991 to 5.9 per cent in 2000 and 7.4 per cent in 2010. Today, the country has around 20 million elderly people. By 2025, this number should rise to 32 million people (IBGE, 2010).

In the last ten years, the absolute growth of Brazil's population has been mainly due to the growth of the adult population, with an increase in the participation of the elderly population (IBGE, 2010). This growth is accompanied by new problems for society, which has few public assistance systems.

According to data from the Situation and Trends Report: Demography and Health (2009) there is an estimate that between 75 and 80 per cent of the population aged 60 and over have at least one chronic condition, which would result in a contingent of 27 million in 2025 and 50 million in 2050. According to the Brazilian Institute of Geography and Statistics (IBGE), the concern should be greater with the elderly population, since only 9.3 per cent of people with chronic non-communicable diseases (CNCD) were reported in the 0-14 age group, while among the elderly this figure reaches 75.5 per cent (IBGE, 2009).

Among the chronic non-communicable diseases (NCDs), cardiovascular diseases, according to the World Health Organisation and the International Society of Hypertension, are responsible for one third of deaths worldwide (Kaplan et al., 2003). According to the European Society of Cardiology, these diseases are responsible for 49 per cent of all deaths and are also the main cause of death in middle-aged and elderly adults in most European countries (Backer et al., 2003). In Brazil, these diseases are responsible for more than 250,000 deaths a year, but systemic arterial hypertension (SAH) is responsible for almost half of them.

The ageing process induces structural changes in the heart and in the vascular properties of the aorta, reducing its functional capacity. In this sense, the individual becomes more susceptible to developing systemic arterial hypertension (SAH), which is the main NCD among the elderly population (Miranda, 2002). In Brazil, it is estimated that more than 60 per cent of the elderly are hypertensive, which can affect 50 per cent of people aged between 60 and 69 and 75 per cent over 70 (SBC, SBH, SBN, 2010).

Several studies have observed that there is a strong correlation between ageing and the prevalence of hypertension. In Canada, studies by Robitaille et al. (2012) found a prevalence of diagnosed hypertension of 43.3 per cent in the 60-64 age group and 62.6 per cent in the 70-74 age group. In India, in Davanagere, Yuvaraj et al. (2010) found a prevalence of 30.5% in the 60-60 age group and 31.3% in the 70+ age group. Similarly, in Brazil, several researchers have identified this correlation: in Campinas/SP, Zaitune et al. (2006) found a prevalence of 51.8% in the 60 and over age group; in Goiânia/GO, Ferreira et al. (2010) found that the prevalence of hypertension was 76.7% in the 60-64 age group and 80.2% in the 70-74 age group.

In order for this situation to change, preventive and therapeutic actions aimed at hypertension, especially in the elderly population, must be exhaustively applied, with an emphasis on modifying lifestyle and controlling and preventing hypertension, even with those who are using drug therapy.

Among these actions, the practice of physical exercise is gaining prominence as an important component for a better quality of life. A study carried out by Church et al. (2001) on 22,167 men over 23 years concluded that the mortality rate was higher among those with lower physical capacity. Blair (1989), when studying physical fitness and mortality in 10,224 men and 3,120 women, observed that individuals with a higher level of physical fitness had lower mortality rates and a delay in all-cause mortality, due to lower rates of cardiovascular disease and cancer in these individuals. Grassi et al. (1992) found lower morbidity and mortality from cardiovascular diseases in physically trained individuals, with clear benefits in the hypertensive subgroup.

Despite the great advances in the study of physical exercise, there is a need for scientific publications that emphasise its influence on the cardiovascular system and the behaviour of blood pressure in elderly hypertensive patients, as well as the specific aspects of its prescription in cardiovascular rehabilitation programmes.

Thus, the aim of this study is to analyse current scientific knowledge about the influence of physical exercise (resistance, aerobic and both in combination) on blood pressure responses and their regulatory mechanisms, as well as the type of exercise most indicated in the literature as a non-pharmacological treatment in elderly hypertensive patients.

CHAPTER 1

HYPERTENSION IN THE ELDERLY

1. INTRODUCTION

As we age, SBP increases linearly from the age of 50, rising linearly until the age of 80 or 90, at around 25 to 35 mmHg, while DBP tends to fall from the age of 55 and increases by 10 to 15 mmHg until the age of 60, before stabilising or gradually reducing (Miranda et al., 2002; Franklin et al., 2005; Oigman et al., 2005).

According to studies carried out by Souza et al. (2007), their data showed that from the age of 60 people had a higher prevalence of isolated systolic hypertension, with a prevalence of 16.4% in individuals aged between 60 and 69 and 24.6% in individuals aged over 70. This is the result of cardiovascular and reflex changes (**Table 1**) resulting from ageing, which can have significant implications for circulatory homeostasis, regardless of whether the individual has pathologies or is healthy (Ferrari et al., 2003).

In the elderly, hypertension comes in two forms: one is the combined form of systolic hypertension (SBP > 140 mmHg) and diastolic hypertension (DBP > 90 mmHg) and the other is isolated systolic hypertension (SBP > 140 mmHg and DBP < 90 mmHg). Isolated systolic hypertension is more common with ageing as a result of structural changes in the arteries (Oigman et al., 2005).

Chart 1: Effects of ageing on important structural and functional characteristics of the cardiovascular system (adapted from Ferrari et al., 2003).

Cardiac changes		Vascular changes	
The weight of the heart	↑	Arterial wall thickness (intima-media)	↑
Dim ensions cardiomyocytes	↑	Sub endothelial collagen	↑
Number of cardiomyocytes	↓	Elastin	↓
Cross-linking collagen	↑	Elastin fragmentation	↑
Ejection fraction		Proteoglycans	↑

Systolic volume	=	Matrix metalloprotease activity	↑
Cardiac output	=	Migration / proliferation of vascular smooth muscle cells into the intima layer.	↑
Start of diastolic filling	=	Arterial distension	↓
End-diastolic filling	↑	Pulse wave speed	↑
Chronotropic response to P-adrenergic stimuli/catecholamines	↓	Total peripheral resistance	↑
Inotropic responsiveness to stimuli / P-adrenergic catecholamines	↓	Endothelial permeability	↑
Inotropic response to digitalis	↓	Endothelial release of nitric oxide	↓
Cardiac output at peak maximal effort	↓	Inflammatory markers/mediators	↑
Lusitropic function	↓	Superoxide dismutase activity	↓
Release of natriuretic peptides	↑	Vasodilation mediated by β-adrenergic	↓

Legend: ↓, decreased↑, increased; =, unchanged.

2. DEFINITION OF HYPERTENSION

According to the VI Brazilian Hypertension Guideline, the definition of systemic arterial hypertension is associated with chronically maintained blood pressure levels equal to or greater than 140 mmHg for systolic blood pressure and/or 90 mmHg for diastolic blood pressure, in adult individuals without the use of antihypertensive therapy. A blood pressure with satisfactory limits is one with levels equal to or lower than 120/80 mmHg and borderline when SBP reaches levels between 130 and 139 mmHg and DBP is 85 to 89 mmHg (SBC, SBH, SBN, 2010).

The classification of hypertension aims to determine groups that have common characteristics in terms of diagnosis, prognosis and treatment, based on scientific data. However, to a certain degree they are contestable, due to the fact that each scientific society has its own classification (Table 1, 2 and 3).

Table 1. Classification of systemic arterial hypertension by the Brazilian Society of Cardiology, the Brazilian Society of Hypertension and the Brazilian Society of Nephrology.

Blood pressure classification

Classification	Systolic pressure (mmHg)	Diastolic pressure (mmHg)
Great	<120	<80
Normal	<130	<85
Borderline	130-139	85-89
Staged hypertension	140-159	90-99
Stage 2 hypertension	160-179	100-109
Stage 3 hypertension	**≥180**	**≥110**
Systolic hypertension isolated	**≥140**	<90
When a patient's systolic and diastolic pressures are in different categories, the higher one should be used to classify blood pressure.		

Source: SBC, SBH, SBN (2010).

Table 2: Classification of SAH by the European Society of Hypertension and the European Society of Cardiology.

Category	Systolic pressure (mmHg)	Diastolic pressure (mmHg)
Optimum pressure	<80	<120
Normal pressure	80-84	120-129
Normal high blood pressure	85-89	130-139
Grade 1 hypertension	90-99	140-159
Grade 2 hypertension	100-109	160-179
Grade 3 hypertension	**≥110**	**≥180**
Isolated systolic hypertension	<90	**≥140**

Source: ESH-European Society of Hypertension.

Table 3: Classification of SAH by the American Heart Association. Blood pressure classification

Blood pressure classification		
Category	**Systolic pressure (mmHg)**	**Diastolic pressure (mmHg)**
Normal pressure	<80	<120
Pre-hypertension	80-89	120-139

Stage 1 hypertension	90-99	140-159
Stage 2 hypertension	**≥110**	**≥160**

Source: American Heart Association.

CHAPTER 2

THE INFLUENCE OF PHYSICAL EXERCISE ON THE PREVENTION AND CONTROL OF SYSTEMIC ARTERIAL HYPERTENSION

1. INTRODUCTION

The hypotensive effect of exercise on hypertensive patients has been the subject of numerous studies over the last few decades, with the reduction in resting diastolic blood pressure after training being the most widely researched. Observational and experimental studies show an inverse association between physical exercise and blood pressure, promoting satisfactory responses for the prevention and control of hypertension, due to autonomic and haemodynamic adjustments (Pescatello et al., 2004; Jannig et al., 2009; Barone et al., 2009; Oliveira et al., 2010).

This is due to the influence that physical exercise has on the body, removing it from its homeostasis, which results in an instantaneous increase in the energy demand of the exercised muscles and, consequently, of the body as a whole. In order to meet the new metabolic demand, various physiological adaptations are required, including those relating to the function of the cardiovascular system during exercise (Brum, 2004).

The regulatory mechanisms responsible for the autonomic and haemodynamic adjustments of the cardiovascular system to exercise and the indices of cardiovascular function limitation are basic aspects related to understanding adaptive functions. Cardiac output, peripheral vascular resistance, or both, as well as changes in serum noradrenaline levels, insulin sensitivity, electrolyte balance, neural and baroreflex mechanisms and vascular structure, are the main regulatory mechanisms that allow the cardiovascular system to operate effectively in the most diverse circumstances (Topol et al., 2005). The physiological adjustments to these mechanisms are made based on metabolic demands, the information from which reaches the brainstem via afferent pathways to the bulbar reticular formation, where the central regulatory neurons are located (Barros et al., 1999).

Haemodynamic mechanisms are more frequently observed in elderly hypertensive patients through a drop in cardiac output; on the other hand, a decrease in peripheral vascular resistance has been analysed in young hypertensive patients, or both, and peripheral vascular resistance and a drop in cardiac output are referred to in various studies as the main mechanism for reducing post-exercise blood pressure in hypertensive patients.

The study carried out by Brandão et al. (2002) showed that the mechanism responsible for the reduction in post-exercise blood pressure was associated with a reduction in cardiac output, since peripheral vascular resistance was not modified in these patients. Hara et al. (1994), in a study of middle-aged hypertensive patients, concluded that the depressant effect of exercise was related to lower peripheral vascular resistance. Rueckert et al. (1996) also observed that after dynamic exercise in hypertensive patients there was a biphasic pattern where initially there was a decrease in peripheral vascular resistance and then, 50 minutes after the end of exercise, the authors observed a decrease in cardiac output.

2. PHYSIOLOGICAL EFFECTS OF PHYSICAL EXERCISE ON BLOOD PRESSURE

The physiological effects of physical exercise on blood pressure can be classified, according to Brandão et al. (2002), as immediate acute, delayed acute and chronic, and this physiological process can be related to both the acute and chronic (training) effects of physical exercise.

In this sense, we can define the acute effects as a response to the effort required of the body, which is directly associated with the exercise session; the immediate acute effects are those that occur in the peri- and post-immediate periods of physical exercise, with an increase in heart rate, pulmonary ventilation and sweating generally associated with the effort; lastly, the late acute effects occur during the first 24 hours following an exercise session and can be identified in the slight reduction in blood pressure levels, especially in hypertensive patients, and in the increase in the number of insulin receptors in muscle cell membranes (I National Consensus on Cardiovascular Rehabilitation, 1997).

For Negrão et al. (2001), from a haemodynamic point of view, the acute effect of physical exercise through a reduction in blood pressure can only be explained by a drop in total peripheral vascular resistance or a reduction in cardiac output.

Chronic effects, also known as long-term physiological adaptations, result from frequent and regular exposure to exercise sessions. Among the most common findings of the chronic effects of exercise are muscle hypertrophy, ventricular hypertrophy, physiological decline, relative resting bradycardia and an increase in maximum oxygen consumption (VO2max), which means the maximum amount of oxygen that the individual can capture from the alveolar air and transport to the tissues via the cardiovascular system and utilise at a cellular level in a unit of time. Consequently, the higher the VO2, the greater the individual's aerobic capacity (I National Consensus on Cardiovascular Rehabilitation, 1997; Bermudes, et al., 2003).

3. POST-EXERCISE BLOOD PRESSURE BEHAVIOUR

The behaviour of post-exercise blood pressure, however, can be modulated by various factors such as the initial level of blood pressure, duration, intensity and type of exercise performed.

In relation to the initial level, the higher this level, the greater the reduction in blood pressure. Bearing in mind the study by Kenney et al. (1993), it can be seen that both in humans and in normotensive and hypertensive rats, post-exercise hypotension is greater in hypertensive subjects. In this study, the reductions induced by maximum intensity exercise in diastolic and systolic blood pressure were, on average, 18 to 20 and 7 to 9 mmHg, respectively, in hypertensive humans and 8 to 10 and 3 to 5 mmHg, respectively, in normotensive humans.

In addition to the initial blood pressure level, the duration of physical exercise is another factor that has been investigated in both normotensive and hypertensive patients, and it has been shown that longer submaximal exercise causes a greater drop in blood pressure and duration than shorter exercise. Overton et al. (1998) observed in a study with hypertensive rats that when the animals ran for 20 minutes, the drop in average blood pressure after 30 minutes of rest was from 158+/-3.6 to 150+/-3.6 mmHg (P less than 0.05). When they ran for 40 minutes on the treadmill, the drop in blood pressure after 30 minutes of rest was 154+/-3.1 to 138+/-3.0 mmHg (P less than 0.05). In the study carried out by Forjaz et al. (1998) with 10 normotensive people, who performed two exercise sessions (25 and 45 minutes) on a cycle ergometer at 50% VO2 peak, they found that mean and diastolic blood pressure decreased significantly post-exercise, as in the 45-minute session.

Considering the intensity of exercise in relation to its hypotensive effect, there are various approaches to its effect in the literature. In this regard, Forjaz et al. (1998) found that the change in blood pressure in normotensive young people who underwent exercise at different intensities (30, 50 and 80% of VO_{2peak}) caused similar hypotension during the recovery period. Veras-Silva et al. (1997), in their study of hypertensive rats with high-intensity (85% VO2 max) and low-intensity (55% VO2 max) exercise training, found that low-intensity exercise lowered blood pressure due to a reduction in cardiac output and a decrease in heart rate. Another researcher, Cunha et al. (2006), in his study comparing the hypotensive effects of

At varying and constant intensities, he found that there was no difference in blood pressure values during the post-exercise recovery period.

Now considering the type of exercise (aerobic, resistance or both performed in combination) that would be most suitable for reducing blood pressure, research has shown that both aerobic and resistance training, and both performed in combination, influence reductions in systolic/diastolic blood pressure in elderly hypertensive patients.

Terra et al. (2008), in a study of 20 sedentary elderly women controlled with antihypertensive medication who underwent a resistance training programme, found that there was a significant reduction in resting systolic blood pressure values.

Sanhueza et al. (2006) also carried out research with sedentary elderly hypertensive women to investigate the influence of aerobic training, and found a significant hypotensive effect on systolic/diastolic blood pressure.

Similarly, Moraes et al. (2011), when investigating the hypotensive effect of a training programme with aerobic and resistance exercises in hypertensive elderly women controlled by antihypertensive medication, found reductions in systolic blood pressure (6 mmHg) and diastolic blood pressure (2 mmHg).

CHAPTER 3

HYPOTENSIVE EFFECT OF AEROBIC EXERCISE IN HYPERTENSION

1. INTRODUCTION

The hypotensive effect of aerobic exercise has been widely studied in view of the important autonomic and haemodynamic changes caused in the cardiovascular system (Brum et al., 2000).

The regular practice of aerobic physical exercise promotes a reduction in blood pressure levels by decreasing peripheral sympathetic activity and cardiac sympathetic tone, and is a determining factor in the decrease in heart rate and, consequently, in cardiac output, favouring a reduction in artery pressure (O'Sullivan et al., 2000).

A systematic review with meta-analysis of 54 longitudinal randomised controlled studies analysing the effect of aerobic exercise on BP seems to prove that this type of exercise reduces SBP (3.8 mmHg) and DBP (2.6 mmHg) on average (Whelton et al., 2002).

Due to a series of studies and reviews confirming the beneficial role of aerobic exercise through its hypotensive effect on hypertensive individuals, many health professionals have been prescribing this type of exercise more effectively and safely as a non-drug treatment for hypertensive individuals classified as having stage I and II hypertension, i.e. mild and moderate (Laterza et al. 2007).

Taylor-Tolbert et al. (2000) showed that a single session of aerobic exercise is enough to reduce blood pressure and can result in a reduced cardiovascular load over a 24-hour period in hypertensive, obese and sedentary elderly men.

Fischer et al. (2002) observed in their study that regular aerobic exercise improved cardiorespiratory parameters in hypertensive elderly women, as well as reducing blood pressure levels. They concluded that aerobic exercise should be indicated for hypertensive patients, due to the similarity of its effort to the effort we make in carrying out daily activities.

Another favourable effect of aerobic exercise was found in the respective studies on hypertensive patients controlled by antihypertensive medication, carried out by Cade et al. (1984) and Oliveira et al. (2010), which was a reduction in the dosage of medication and in others the interruption of all medication, reducing financial costs and the side effects that medication entails.

Bearing in mind that the beneficial effects of physical training are transient and reversible, and may disappear with a reduction or lack of exercise, Kokkinos et al. (1997) suggest that hypertensive patients without clinical contraindications to exercise should be encouraged to take part in a programme of aerobic exercise of light to moderate intensity, even when resting blood pressure is controlled with drugs.

Numerous beneficial effects have been mentioned above, however, there are caveats to its prescription for hypertensive patients or people with heart problems. The Brazilian Society of Hypertension (2006) emphasises that in stage III hypertensive patients, aerobic activities with an intensity of more than 70% of VO2 max can be harmful and are contraindicated. However, it should be started as soon as blood pressure is controlled, with careful monitoring in relation to the general principles of physical exercise.

These principles are made up of three distinct periods: warm-up, aerobic phase and return to calm, which ensure the prescription of exercises in hypertension, especially in the elderly population. These rules are recommended in order to avoid harmful increases in blood pressure levels in the population being treated (Chobanian et al., 2003).

2. ANALYSIS OF AEROBIC EXERCISE PROGRAMMES FOR ELDERLY HYPERTENSIVE PATIENTS

The table below summarises aerobic training programmes that have investigated the influence of physical exercise on elderly hypertensive men and women. The studies were selected from electronic databases: MEDLINE (1966 to the present), PubMed (1950 to the present), LILACS (1982 to the present), SciELO (1998 to the present).

Studies investigating the influence of physical exercise on hypertensive elderly men and women were selected. The search and selection of articles was carried out using the following procedures: keywords in Portuguese, English and Spanish in the following sequence - hypertension (hypertension, hypertensión); physical exercise (physical exercise, ejercicio físico); elderly (idoso, ansiano); aerobic exercise (ejercicio aeróbico).

Randomised controlled trials (RCTs) or quasi-RCTs (quasi-random distribution), case studies that carried out interventions involving physical exercise in elderly hypertensive patients and previous systematic review studies were included in this research.

The studies that met the inclusion criteria were analysed independently by the two reviewers in order to obtain the following information: authors, year of publication, study design, participants, intervention used, outcome of key variables.

Table 4 - Aerobic training programmes based on scientific studies

Study/Country	Participants	Training programme	Results
Fisher et al., 2002. Brazil.	Elderly women with mild primary hypertension who practised regular physical activity. Average age: 60. N= 2 Case study 1 (Makes use of the pen blocker) Case study II (No beta blocker)	Duration and frequency: Study 1 -13 months and study 11-10 months. 3 times a week, lasting 1 hour. Intensity: 60 to 85% VO2 of maximum frequency. Training programme: 10 minutes of warm-up stretching; 30 minutes of aerobic activity divided between treadmill and stationary bike; 15 minutes of low-load localised aerobic activity using resources such as a ball, stick and low-load weight and 5 minutes of relaxation.	Case study 1 - Reduction in blood pressure both at rest and at peak Case study II - Reduction in blood pressure both at rest and at peak.
Sanhueza	Elderly people with	Duration: 10 weeks	The EG saw a

et al. 2006. Chile.	hypertension and sedentary lifestyles. N= 37 Exercise group (GE) = 18 Control Group (CG) =19	Exercise group (EG) Frequency and intensity: 3 times a week, with an approximate 70-80 % VO2 max. Programme: 2 weeks of global conditioning, with calisthenic exercises for 50-60 minutes. 8-week clinical programme: 15 minutes of calisthenic exercise (warm-up), 30 minutes of aerobic exercise (walking and jogging), 15 minutes of calisthenic exercise (cool-down). Control Group: no intervention	significant decrease: 'Systolic blood pressure (7 mmHg) *Diastolic blood pressure (5 mmHg)
Lee et al., 2007. China.	Elderly people with mild to moderate hypertension - use of anti-inflammatory medication hypertensive N= 202 Intervention group (n=102) Control group (n=100)	Duration: 6 months Intervention group: Community-based walking. Control group: Primary health care.	The difference in the average change in systolic blood pressure was 15.4 mm Hg for the intervention group and 8.4 mm Hg for the control group. The mean difference between the two groups was -7.0 mm Hg.

In summary, when analysing the results of the programmes on systolic blood pressure (SBP), reductions in blood pressure were seen where the intervention adopted in the programmes used aerobic exercise (Fisher et al., 2002; Sanhueza et al., 2006; Lee et al., 2007). The reduction in SBP is a positive result in the elderly hypertensive population, given that Systolic Arterial Hypertension is an important modifiable cardiovascular risk factor and that the physiological changes resulting from arterial ageing make individuals more prone to developing it.

In the study carried out by Sanhueza et al (2006), the participants were randomised into a control group and an experimental group. The protocol for the experimental group consisted of aerobic exercise at an intensity of 70 to 80 per cent of maximum oxygen consumption (VO_{2max}), three times a day, lasting 60 minutes per session for ten weeks. The control group only undertook a regular physical activity programme. When comparing blood pressure values between the groups, the experimental group achieved a significant decrease in SBP and DBP.

Similarly, Fisher et al. (2002), in a case study of two hypertensive elderly women, carried out an aerobic exercise programme at an intensity of 60 to 85% of VO_{2max}, three times a week, lasting 60 minutes each session, for thirteen months. They concluded that there was a reduction in resting systolic and diastolic blood pressure.

When we compare the studies, we can see that there is a similarity between the blood pressure responses in the significant reduction of SBP and DBP and the exercise protocols (intensity and duration of the session).

The protocols of the aforementioned studies followed the recommendations of the Brazilian Hypertension Guidelines (2006) and the American College of Sports Medicine (2004), which recommend that aerobic exercise should be carried out at an intensity of 50 to 70 per cent of maximum oxygen consumption, three or more sessions a week, lasting 30 to 60 minutes for each session.

Another form of aerobic exercise featured in this chapter is walking; based on self-efficacy theory, Lee et al. (2007) carried out a six-month intervention programme with elderly hypertensive patients using walking. The participants were randomised into an intervention group and a control group. The intervention group was instructed to walk regularly, increasing the frequency and time spent. Initially, a pedometer was provided to make it easier for the participants to walk regularly. Both the control group and the intervention group took part in the primary health care programme. At six-month follow-up, the average change in systolic blood pressure resulted in a decrease of 15.4 mmHg and 8.4 mmHg in the intervention group and control group, respectively. The difference in mean change between the two groups was 7.0 mmHg. However, no differences were observed in the groups' diastolic blood pressure. With regard to the self-efficacy exercise scores, the intervention group was more likely to answer that they had started walking more, resulting in an improvement in the scores.

Analysing the studies, we can see that regular walking is one of the forms of non-pharmacological treatment for the elderly. The reduction in systolic blood pressure found in the study is a fact of great relevance in the elderly, since we assume that from the age of 50 SBP increases linearly (Miranda et al., 2002).

According to Matsudo (2008), walking is one of the most recommended activities because it is low impact and can be performed at different intensities by elderly hypertensive patients, bringing numerous health benefits.

CHAPTER 4

HYPOTENSIVE EFFECT OF RESISTANCE EXERCISE IN HYPERTENSION

1.INTRODUCTION

Resistance exercise consists of local muscle work carried out using various types of overload, such as weights, weight training, etc.

In this context, it is important to recognise the importance of the use of equipment, specific machines, elastic bands, body mass or any other form of equipment that aids in the development of muscular strength, power or endurance (Bermudes et al., 2004).

This type of exercise can be carried out with moderate loads and frequent repetitions, with pauses between executions, characterising it as a discontinuous effort (Conley et al., 2001). During its execution, a significant increase in cardiovascular responses can be expected, especially if performed until fatigue (MacDougall et al., 1985).

The resistance of each exercise can be related to a certain percentage of the highest possible load to be mobilised in a single maximum repetition (1-RM) or related to a stipulated number of maximum repetitions (American College of Sports Medicine, 2002).

Maximum dynamic strength can be represented by the one repetition maximum (1RM) test. This test assesses the greatest load that can be lifted or overcome, alternating between concentric and eccentric muscle contractions (MacDougall et al., 1991). Standardising strength and endurance reduces the variation in test results in order to achieve the proposed objectives.

The hypotensive effect of resistance exercise can be influenced by variations in intensity, resting blood pressure level, muscle mass involved and the body segment used in the exercise. In relation to the muscle mass involved, MacDonald et al. (2000), in their study with hypertensive patients, concluded that the mass of the working muscle does not directly affect the magnitude of post-exercise hypotension, but can influence the duration of the response, suggesting that the central mechanism or the low vascular response is responsible for post-exercise hypotension.

In the study carried out by Lizardo and Simões (2005) with trained normotensive individuals, it was found that the sessions involving greater muscle mass (lower limbs) had a more significant and longer-lasting hypotensive effect than the upper limb session.

However, Terra et al. (2008), in a study of hypertensive elderly women, using the alternating segment training method, with randomised exercises involving lower and upper limb muscle mass, showed that there was a reduction in resting systolic blood pressure, while there was no reduction in diastolic blood pressure.

In the research by Cunha et al. (2012), it was also found that the training group showed a reduction in both resting diastolic blood pressure and mean arterial pressure; on the other hand, the light resistance training group showed a reduction in mean arterial pressure, with a tendency towards a reduction in diastolic blood pressure in hypertensive elderly women controlled by antihypertensive medication.

Finally, it is worth noting the official position of the American College of Sports Medicine, which stresses the importance of including resistance training in a programme for the prevention, treatment and control of hypertension (Pescatello et al., 2004).

2. ANALYSIS OF RESISTANCE EXERCISE PROGRAMMES FOR ELDERLY HYPERTENSIVE PATIENTS

The table below summarises aerobic training programmes that have investigated the influence of physical exercise on elderly hypertensive men and women. The studies were selected from electronic databases: MEDLINE (1966 to the present), PubMed (1950 to the present), LILACS (1982 to the present), SciELO (1998 to the present).

Studies investigating the influence of physical exercise on hypertensive elderly men and women were selected. The search and selection of articles was carried out using the following procedures: keywords in Portuguese, English and Spanish in the following sequence - hypertension (hypertension, hypertensión); physical exercise (physical exercise, ejercicio físico); elderly (idoso, ansiano); resistance exercise (resistance exercise, ejercicio resistencia).

Randomised controlled trials (RCTs) or quasi-RCTs (quasi-random distribution), case studies that carried out interventions involving physical exercise in elderly hypertensive patients and previous systematic review studies were included in this research.

The studies that met the inclusion criteria were analysed independently by the two reviewers in order to obtain the following information: authors, year of publication, study design, participants, intervention used, outcome of key variables.

Table 5: Effect of resistance exercise on blood pressure in elderly hypertensive patients.

Study/Country	Participants	Training programme	Results
Krinski et *al, 2008.* Brazil	Elderly women with stage 1 hypertension. Mean age = 63.75 ± 3.70 years N= 24	Duration and Frequency: 1 weight circuit session, with 8 stations, 3x12 repetitions. Intensity: 50% of 1 RM -Training programme : Leg press 45° , squat, extension table, knee bend, bench press, *pulley* pull, biceps curl and triceps *pulley.*	Statistically significant reduction in DBP for the resting condition.
Terra et *al,* 2008. Brazil	Elderly sedentary hypertensive women controlled with anti-hypertensive medication. Average age > 60 years. N= 52 Resistance training group = 23 Control group = 29	**Resistance training group (GTR)** Duration and Frequency: 12 weeks, 3 times a week on alternate days in 3 sets of 12, 10 and 8 repetitions. Intensity: 4 initial weeks, the intensity was 60% of 1-RM, 4 subsequent weeks 70% of 1-rM and 4 weeks 80% of 1-rM. -Training programme : Pull-up back, knee extension, bench press, abductor chair, knee flexion, shoulder abduction with dumbbell, free standing calf raises, abdominals, trunk extension and 45° leg press. **Control group**: no exercise	Training The reduction was 10.5 mmHg for SBP without reducing DBP. Control group: No difference.
Janning et *al., 2009.* Brazil	Elderly people without previous experience in resistance training for hypertensive patients controlled with	Duration and Frequency: 7 days, with an interval of at least 48 hours between each protocol. Intensity: 3 x 12 RM, with an interval of two to three minutes between each set of exercises. After each protocol, blood pressure was	There was no reduction in DBP in P1 and P2. At P3, there was an average reduction in SBP (11.3 ± 9.1) and DBP (4.4 ± 4.5

	antihypertensive medication. Average age = 62.1 ± 3.1 years N= 8 (4 men and 4 women).	checked at 10-minute intervals up to 60 minutes post-exercise. Training programme: **Protocol 1** (P1) - Order of execution: 1) /eg press 90°; 2) knee extension; 3) knee flexion; 4) bench press; 5) anterior high pull; and 6) high row. **Protocol 2** (P2) - Inverse: Performing the three upper limb exercises first, followed by the three lower limb exercises. **Protocol 3 (**P3) - Interspersed: One exercise for the upper limbs with one for the lower limbs.	mmHg).
Costa et al., 2010. Brazil	Trained and untrained hypertensive elderly women using antihypertensive medication. Average age = 66 ± 4 years. N= 15 Trained group (GT) = 06. Grou p no trained (GNT) = 09 weekly.	Duration and Frequency: 2 randomised sessions, one experimental (SE) and the other control (SC), with a 48-hour interval between sessions. Intensity: 40 min of exercises with dynamic weights, performed in 2 sets of 10 to 15 maximum repetitions. Training programme: • Bench press, rowing convergent, scott curl, pulley triceps, extension table, flexor table and adductor chair. • The recovery interval between sets was one minute and between exercises was 2 minutes. During this period, BP was measured at minutes 0, 15, 30, 45 and 60.	An exer cise session with weights can reduce post-exercise blood pressure.
Canuto et al., 2011. Brazil	Wome n with diag nosis systemic arterial hypertension with the use of anti-hypertensive medication. **Average age £** 60. N = 32 Light load group (G1) = 16 High intensity load group (G2) = 16	Duration: 3 sessions of resistance exercise, followed by systolic and diastolic blood pressures measured every 10 minutes for 1 hour. Intensity: G1 participants performed 2x16 repetitions with half the 8RM load and G2 participants performed 2 x 8 repetitions with an 8RM load. Training programme: - The exercises were always performed in the following order: leg press, bench press, knee extension with extension chair, front pull, knee flexion on flexor table, lateral elevation of upper limbs with dumbbells, hip abduction with cross over and barbell curls. -	It did not result in post-exercise hypotension.
Oliveira et al., 2011. Brazil	Men with stage I hypertension, practising physical activity. No use of anti-hypertensive medication with medical clearance	Duration and Frequency: 2 sessions with a 48-hour interval between sessions. Intensity: Two training sessions at 80% and 100% of 10 RM During the activity and up to 24 hours afterwards, the subjects were monitored by ambulatory blood pressure monitoring	Occurrence of PEH for SBP, DBP, being significantly hig her in the 80% intensity

	for 2 weeks prior to starting the experiment. Average age = 6.0 ± 4.4 years. N = 10	(ABPM). Systolic and diastolic blood pressure and pulse pressure were assessed. Training programme: - Leg press 45°, Bench press on the Smith Machine.	Work smaller intensities, such as 80% of 10RM may be more efficient in these reductions.
Park et al., 2011. South Korea	Elderly people with diagnosis for more than a year, controlled by anti-inflammatory medication hypertension. N= 45 Group intervention (n=18) Control group (n=22)	Duration and frequency: 12 weeks, twice a week **Intervention group:** Training programme: • Warm-up: 15 minutes light stretching, 1 set. • Main exercise: Push-ups, extension, front raise, side shoulder raise, biceps flexion, triceps extension, elbow extension, shoulder extension, seated row, front shoulder raise, leg press, squat, hip extension, straight abdominal, pelvic lift, lower abdominal. 40 minutes, 15-25 repetitions, 2-3 sets. • Warming up: 5 minutes light stretching, 1 set. **Control group**: Health education and individual counselling.	The intervention group showed a significantly greater reduction in systolic blood pressure.
Cunha et *al.,* 2012. Brazil	Elderly hypertensive women, controlled by anti-inflammatory medication hypertension. N = 16 Group moderate resistance training (G1) = 09 Group light resistance training (G2) = 07	Duration and frequency: 8 weeks, 3 times a week on alternate days, in the afternoon. Intensity: **G1** performed 2x8 repetitions with an 8RM load and G2 performed 2 x 16 repetitions with half the 8RM load. Training programme: -The exercises carried out were respectively leg press, bench press, knee extension, front pull, knee flexion, shoulder abduction, unilateral hip abduction with cross over and barbell curl.	Training moderate resistance promoted reductions in DBP. Training resistedlight caused a tendency to reduce DBP.

In summary, with resistance exercise, studies have shown a reduction in blood pressure (Janning et al., 2009; Costa et al., 2010; Oliveira et al., 2011), systolic blood pressure (Terra et al., 2008) and diastolic blood pressure (Krinski et al., 2008).

The knowledge acquired in recent decades suggests that after a single session of resistance exercise, blood pressure levels decrease and remain below pre-exercise levels. Based on Table 6, the studies evaluated the acute cardiovascular effects of resistance exercise in relation to systolic and diastolic blood pressure.

Studies carried out by Costa et al. (2010) in a resistance exercise training session with a group of trained (weight training) and untrained (stretching) elderly women indicated a decline in SBP after exercise in both groups, but more consistently in the untrained (stretching) group. The weight-trained group showed a reduction in SBP only after 30 minutes of recovery, while the untrained group showed a reduction after 15 minutes and 60 minutes of post-exercise monitoring. With regard to DBP, the hypotensive effect of the weight training session was only observed in the untrained group (stretching), at 15 and 30 minutes of recovery.

In contrast to the previous exercise, Krinski et al. (2008) in a study with elderly hypertensive women (stage I) and involving a session of resistance exercise, found that there was a significant decrease only in DBP. These results are similar to those of Cunha et al. (2012), carried out with hypertensive elderly women, and differ only in the duration of the programme, which was eight weeks, concluding that moderate resistance training promoted reductions in DBP.

However, Oliveira et al. (2011), when carrying out two sessions of resistance exercise with elderly (male) hypertensive individuals (stage I) who practised physical activity, found that a single session of RE carried out at different intensities (80% and 100% of 10RM) promoted PEH in elderly hypertensive individuals (stage I), leading to changes in the average classification category of elderly hypertensive individuals, from pre-hypertension to normal, reducing the risk of cardiovascular events. However, the authors emphasise that working at intensities of 80% of 10 RM can be effective in these reductions.

In contrast to this study, Canuto et al. (2011) carried out an intervention in women diagnosed with systemic arterial hypertension and found that a sequence of resistance exercises lasting three training sessions did not result in post-exercise hypotension in elderly hypertensive women. This evidence is due to the lack of significant differences in systolic and diastolic blood pressure in the groups after light and high intensity exercise.

There are several reasons why resistance exercise did not produce similar results between the studies. One of the reasons can be attributed in part to the characteristics of the sample, i.e. the fact that it was made up of elderly hypertensive patients. It is well known that with ageing, the cardiovascular system undergoes changes in its ability to adapt to and recover from exercise, with the differences between age and the reaction to submaximal and maximal exercise being more noticeable. Thus, in addition to the tendency to maintain high BP related to genetics and the environment, the ageing factor seems to contribute to maintaining high BP (Cardoso et al., 2010).

Janning et al. (2009), when analysing the influence of the order in which resistance exercises were performed on post-exercise hypotension in controlled hypertensive elderly subjects, randomly subjected their sample to three different protocols. These were carried out over a period of seven days, starting on the day the 12 RM loads were determined, with an interval of at least 48 hours between each protocol. In protocol 1 (P1) the exercises were organised in the following order: 1) 90° *leg press*; 2) knee extension; 3) knee flexion; 4) bench press; 5) anterior high pull; and 6) high row. The sequence of exercises shows that first all the exercises were for the IM and then all for the MS. In protocol 2 (P2) the situation was reversed, with the three upper limb exercises performed first, followed by the three lower limb exercises. Protocol 3 (P3) was organised in such a way as to intersperse one upper limb exercise with another for the lower limbs.

The authors concluded that P1, at the end of the session with three upper limb exercises, showed no significant drop in blood pressure. When observing P2, it can be seen that PEH occurred at times, suggesting that this drop in blood pressure was due to the fact that the inactive muscles (IM) were relatively smaller compared to the active muscles (IM), since the last three exercises were performed for IM. However, P3 proved to be extremely effective in producing PEH through exercises performed with alternating limbs.

However, the appropriate and well-supervised prescription of resistance exercise is of great importance to guarantee the effectiveness of the programme in the prevention, treatment and control of hypertension (Pescatello et al., 2004).

According to Williams (2007), health institutions such as the American College of Sports Medicine (ASCM) and the American Heart Association (AHA) have started to recommend resistance training as a complement to aerobic training for individuals with cardiovascular problems, especially women and the elderly.

3. ANALYSIS OF AEROBIC EXERCISE PROGRAMMES ASSOCIATED WITH RESISTANCE TRAINING FOR ELDERLY HYPERTENSIVE PATIENTS

The table below summarises aerobic training programmes that have investigated the influence of physical exercise on elderly hypertensive men and women. The studies were selected from electronic databases: MEDLINE (1966 to the present), PubMed (1950 to the present), LILACS (1982 to the present), SciELO (1998 to the present).

Studies investigating the influence of physical exercise on hypertensive elderly men and women were selected. The search and selection of articles was carried out using the following procedures: keywords in Portuguese, English and Spanish in the following sequence - hypertension (hypertension, hypertensión); physical exercise (physical exercise, ejercicio físico); elderly (idoso, ansiano); aerobic and resistance exercise (ejercicio aeróbico y de resistencia).

Randomised controlled trials (RCTs) or quasi-RCTs (quasi-random distribution), case studies that carried out interventions involving physical exercise in elderly hypertensive patients and previous systematic review studies were included in this research.

The studies that met the inclusion criteria were analysed independently by the two reviewers in order to obtain the following information: authors, year of publication, study design, participants, intervention used, outcome of key variables.

Table 6: Effect of combined aerobic and resistance exercise on blood pressure in elderly hypertensive patients.

Study/ Country	Participants	Intervention	Results
Barros et al., 2008. Brazil	Elderly people with stage I hypertension, without the use of antipsychotics. hypertension, two weeks before starting the programme. Average age: 66.5 ± 4 years (61 to 79) N= 45 Study Group (SG) = 24 (five men) Control Group (CG) = 21 (four men)	Duration: 6 months **Study Group (SG)**: Guidance for non-pharmacological treatment and supervised physical activity. Frequency and duration: 3 sessions a week, each lasting 1 hour. Training programme: • 30 minutes of aerobic activity on bicycles and treadmills, with the goal of maintaining a heart rate between 60 and 75 per cent of the maximum heart rate (MHR) reached at peak effort in the ET. • 30 minutes of flexibility and weight-bearing activities (resistance exercises) with loads of 40% to 60% of the maximum repetition (RM) in 3 sets of 10 repetitions. **Control Group (CG)**: They received guidance for non-pharmacological treatment.	Supervised physical activity was more effective in maintaining blood pressure control in elderl y people with stage I hypertension (SG) when compared to the control group.
Rêgo et al., 2011. Brazil	Sweethe arts se dentary hypertensive women undergoing pharmacological treatment. **Average age > 60** years. Experimental Group (EG) = 26 Control Group (CG) = 15	Duration and Frequency: 18 weeks (35 sessions), twice a week. **Experimental Group** - Intensity: Low or moderate, according to Borg's subjective scale. Training programme: • **10' of stretching exercises;** • **35' ofaerobic endurance** (walking) and muscular (localised exercises with 2 sets of 10 repetitions); • **10' stretching with 5'** relaxation. **Control Group** - No exercise	Average decrease in SBP of 9.615mmHg and DBP of 1.25mmHg.
Morae s et al., 2012 Brazil	Elderly people with hypertension controlled with antiplatelet medic ation hypertension N= 44	Duration and frequency: 12 weeks, with two sessions a week. Intensity: Moderate, according to the Subjective Effort Scale. Training programme: - Sessions lasting approximately 60 minutes consisting of a warm-up period, followed by stretching (±10 minutes); a main part, lasting 35 to 40 minutes, consisting of around 20 minutes of walking and the rest dedicated to dancing, interspersed with strength exercises with dumbbells and sticks; finally, **a "return to calm" activity, with** stretching for 10 minutes.	It was reduced: Blood pressure systolic (6 mm Hg) Blood pressure diastolic (2 mm Hg)

The studies used aerobic exercise combined with resistance training as a training programme, with the aim of assessing its hypotensive effect on blood pressure. However, none of the studies evaluated the acute effect of this type of exercise, which lasted from twelve weeks to six months, with a frequency of two to three sessions per week.

Barroso et al. (2008) assessed men and women aged over 60 with arterial hypertension (stage I) who had not taken antihypertensive drugs in the two weeks prior to the intervention. The authors observed a slight reduction in both SBP and DBP values after six months of intervention. They concluded that there was a decrease, without statistical significance, in systolic and diastolic blood pressure levels, i.e. the exercise programme resulted in the same blood pressure levels after six months without the use of hypotensive medication.

However, Rêgo et al. (2011), with sedentary hypertensive elderly women taking antihypertensive medication, underwent an aerobic exercise programme combined with resistance training for eighteen weeks, with two sessions a week, each lasting sixty minutes. They found that there were changes in systolic and diastolic blood pressure levels, with significant reductions over eighteen weeks.

Similarly, Moraes et al. (2011), in their research, observed that this type of combination of physical exercise, in which the authors subjected elderly hypertensive patients controlled by medication, for twelve weeks, with two weekly sessions, lasting sixty minutes each session. They concluded that this combination of exercise was capable of reducing blood pressure levels, as well as increasing muscle strength, aerobic capacity and balance, with repercussions on improving functional capacity.

It should be noted that the studies by Barroso et al. (2008), Rêgo et al. (2011) and Moraes et al. (2011) are similar in terms of sample, type of exercise, duration and frequency. However, the study by Barroso et al. (2008) differs from the others in terms of sample and results. With regard to the results, the hypotensive effect after exercise occurred for both SBP and DBP, but without statistical significance; with regard to the sample, the elderly were not using antihypertensive drugs, so it was possible to determine the isolated effect of exercise.

However, the studies carried out by Rêgo et al. (2011) and Moraes et al. (2011) showed a significant reduction in blood pressure levels. It should be noted that due to the use of antihypertensive medication, it was not possible to determine the isolated effect of exercise, but only to observe the effect of combining drug therapy with physical exercise.

Similar to the studies mentioned above, authors such as Fisher et al. (2002), Lee et al. (2007), Moraes et al. (2011), Park et al. (2011), Rêgo et al. (2011), Cunha et al. (2012), had reductions in blood pressure levels, although it was not possible to determine the isolated effect of exercise, due to the use of antihypertensive medication used by the sample.

However, there are some factors such as the characteristics of the population studied, the pathophysiology and different stages of hypertension, pharmacodynamics and pharmacokinetics, which seem to influence the internal validity of the studies, as well as the methodological quality of the research.

CHAPTER 5

CONCLUSION

Despite the small number of studies included in this review analysing the influence of physical exercise on elderly hypertensive patients, the main results of the research seem to indicate that aerobic exercise generates significant decreases in SBP and DBP levels, both at rest and on exertion, after a period of training.

Resistance exercises performed three or two times a week at moderate intensity were found to reduce blood pressure in elderly hypertensive patients, especially systolic blood pressure.

In relation to the combination of physical exercises, it was also possible to see that the use of a physical training programme based on aerobic exercises associated with resistance exercise (circuit with weights) resulted in significant reductions in systolic and diastolic blood pressure, as well as increasing muscle strength, aerobic capacity and balance, with repercussions on improving functional capacity, which was superior to performing the exercise modalities in isolation, which confirms the guidelines of the VI Brazilian Guidelines for Arterial Hypertension (2010).

Considering these aspects, we can say that the different types of exercise discussed in this review seem to have a positive influence on blood pressure levels in elderly hypertensive patients (reduction). As a result, their prescription should be recommended whenever possible in the elderly hypertensive population (stage I and II), due to the benefits that physical exercise causes both in the cardiovascular system and in other systems of the body.

With regard to the methodological rigour and clarity of the studies included in this review, after a careful assessment of their methodological quality, there was a lack of information regarding the interventions used and the methods reported by the researchers.

Finally, it is worth mentioning the relevance of carrying out this systematic review due to the scarcity of studies looking at the influence of the hypotensive response of physical exercise in different exercise programmes in the elderly hypertensive population.

BIBLIOGRAPHY

Akobeng, A. K. (2005). Understanding randomised controlled trials. *Arch. Dis. Child.* 90(8), 840-4.

Alves, L. C., Leimann, B. C. Q., Vasconcelos, M. E. L., Carvalho, M. S., Vasconcelos, A. G. G., Fonseca, T. C. O., Lebrão, M. L., Laurenti, R. (2007). The influence of chronic diseases on the functional capacity of the elderly in the municipality of São Paulo, Brazil. *Cadernos de Saúde Pública*, Rio de Janeiro, 23(8),1924-1930.

American College of Sports Medicine (2004). Position Stand: Exercise and Hypertension. *Medicine & Science in Sports & Exercise*, 36(3), 533-553.

American College of Sports Medicine (2002). Progression models in resistance training for healthy adults. *Med. Sci. Sports.* Exerc.2(34), 364-80.

Backer, G., Ambrosioni, E., Borch-Jonhsen, K. (2003). European guidelines on cardiovascular disease prevention in clinical practise. Third Joint Task Force of European and other Societies on Cardiovascular Disease Prevention in Clinical Practise. *Eur. J. Cardiovascular Prev. Rehab.* 03(10) (Suppl 1): S1- S78.

Barone, B. B., Wang, N. Y., Bacher, A. C., Stewart, K. J. (2009). Decreased exercise blood pressure in older adults after exercise training: contributions of increased fitness and decreased fatness. *Br. J. Sports* Med.43(1), 52-6.

Barros Neto, T. L., César, M. C., Tebexreni, A. S. (1999). Exercise physiology. In Ghorayeb, N., Barros, T.L. (Ed). *Exercise. Physiological preparation, medical assessment, special and preventive aspects* (pp. 3- 13).São Paulo: Atheneu.

Barroso, W. K. S., Jardim, P. C. B. V., Vitorino, P. V., Bittencourt, A., Miquetichuc, F.(2008). Influence of programmed physical activity on blood pressure in elderly hypertensive patients under non-pharmacological treatment. *Rev Assoc Med Bras.* 54(4), 328-33.

Bermudes, A. M. L. M., Vassallo, D. V., Vasquez, E. C., Lima, E. G. (2004). Ambulatory blood pressure monitoring in normotensive individuals submitted to two single exercise sessions: resistance and aerobic.*Arq. Bras. Cardiologia,*82(1), 57-64.

Blair, S. N., Kohl, H. W., Paffenbarger Jr., R. S., Clark, D. G., Cooper, K. H., Gibbons, L.W. (1989). Physical fitness and all-cause mortality. *JAMA* (262), 2395-401.

Brandão, R. M. U. P., Alves, M. J. N. N., Braga, A. M. F. W., et al. (2002). Post exercise blood pressure reduction in elderly hypertensive patients. J. *Am. Coll. Cardiol.* 39(4), 676-82.

Brandão, A. P., Brandão, A. A., Magalhães, M. E. C., Pozzan, R. (2003). Epidemiology of arterial hypertension. Rev. Soc. Cardiol.,13(1),7-19.

Brum, P. C., Forjaz, C. L. M., Tinucci, T., Negrão, C. E. (2004). Rev. Paul. Educ. Phys., 18,21-31.

Brum, P. C., Silva, G. J., Moreira, E. D., et al. (2000). Exercise training increases baroreceptor gain sensitivity in normal and hypertensive rats. *Hypertension,* 36(6), 1018-22.

Cade, R., Mars, D., Wagemaker, H., et al. (1984). Effect aerobic exercise training on patients with systemic arterial hypertension. Am. J. *Med.,77,* 78590.

Canuto, P. M. B. C., Nogueira, I. D. B., Cunha, E. S., Ferreira, G. M. H., Mendonça, K. M. P. P., Costa, F. A., Nogueira, P. A. M. S. (2011). Influence of Resistance Training Performed at Different Intensities and Same Work Volume on the Blood Pressure of Elderly Hypertensive Women. Rev *Bras Med* Esporte, 17(4), 246-249.

Cardoso Jr., C. G., Gomides, R.S., Queiroz, A.C.C., Pinto, L.G., Lobo, F.S., Tinucci, T., et al. (2010). Acute and chronic effects of aerobic and resistance exercise on ambulatory blood pressure. Clinics, 65, 317-25.

Chobanian, A.V., Bakris, G. L., Black, H. R., Cushman, W. C., Green, L. A., Izzo, J. L. Jr., et al. (2003). Seventh report of the joint National Committee on Prevention, Detection, Evaluation, and Treatment of High Blood Pressure.Hypertension, 42(6), 1206-52.

Chobanian, A.V., Bakris, G. L., Black, H. R., Cushman, W. C., Green, L. A., Izzo, J. L. Jr., et al. (2003). The Seventh Report of the Joint National Committee on Prevention, Detection, Evaluation.JAMA, 289(19), 2560-2571.

Chruch, T.S., et al. (2001). Usefulness of cardiorespiratory fitness as a predictor of allcause and cardiovascular disease mortality in men with systemic hypertension. Am J Cardiol. 88, 651-6.

Conley, M. S., Rozenek, R. (2001). National Strength and Conditioning Association position statement: Health aspects of resistance exercise and training. Strength Cond. J., 23, 9-23.

Costa, L. O., Moseley, A. M., Sherrington, C., Maher, C. G., Herbert, R. D., Elkins, M. R. (2010). Core journals that publish clinical trials of physical therapy interventions. Phys Ther., 90(11), 1631-40.

Cunha, G. A., Rios, A. C. S., Moreno, J. R., Braga, P. L., Campbell, C. S. G.,

Simões, G. H., Denadai, M. L. D. R. (2006). Post-exercise hypotension in hypertensive patients undergoing aerobic exercise of varying intensities and constant intensity exercise. Rev. Bras. Med. Esporte, 12(6), 313-317.

Cunha E. S, Miranda, P. A., Nogueira, S., Costa, E. C., Silva, E. P., Ferreira, G. M. H. (2012). Resistance training intensities and blood pressure in hypertensive elderly women - a pilot study. Rev *Bras Med Esporte,* 18(6), 373376.

Brazilian Hypertension Guidelines, V. Brazilian Society of Hypertension; Brazilian Society of Cardiology; Brazilian Society of Nephrology, 2006.

Fagard, R. H., Cornelissen, V. A. (2007). Effect of exercise on blood pressure control in hypertensive patients. *Eur. J. Cardiovasc. Prev. Rehabil.*, 14, 12-7.

Ferrari, A., Radaelli, A., Centola, M. (2003). Aging and the cardiovascular system. J *Appl. Physiol,* 95, 591-2597.

Fisher MM. (2001). The effect of resistance exercise on recovery blood pressure in normotensive and borderline hypertensive women. *J. Strength. Cond. Res.*, 15, 210-216.

Forjaz, C. L.M., Matsudaira, Y., Rodrigues, F. B., Nunes, N., Negrão, C.E. (1998). Post-exercise changes in blood pressure, heart rate and rate pressure product at different exercise intensities in normotensive humans. *Braz. J. Med. Biol. Res.,* 31, 1247 - 255

Forjaz, C. L. M., Santaella, D. F., Rezende, L. O., Barretto, A. C. P., Negrão, C. E. (1998). Exercise duration determines the magnitude and duration of post-exercise hypotension. *Arq. Bras. Cardiol.,*70, 99-104.

Franklin, S. S., Pio. J. R., Wong, N. D., Larson, M. G., Leip, E. P., Vasan, R. S., Levy, D. (2005). Predictors of new-onset diastolic and systolic hypertension: the Framingham Heart Study. *Circulation,111,1121-27.*

Grassi, G., Seravalle, G., Calhoun, D.C., Boela, G.B., Mancia, G. (1992).Physical exercise in essential hypertension.*Chest,* 101, 3125-45.

Hagberg, J. M., Montain, S. J., Martin, W. H. (1989). Effect of exercise training in 60 to 69 year old persons with essential hypertension.*Am. J. Cardiol.,*64, 348-54.

Hara, K., Floras, J.S. (1994). Influence of naloxone on muscle sympathetic nerve activity, systemic and calf haemodynamics and ambulatory blood pressure after exercise in mild essential hypertension. *J. Hypertens.*,13, 44761.

Huang, G., Shi, X., Davis-Brezette, J. A., Osness, W. H. (2005). Resting heart rate changes after endurance training in older adults: a meta-analysis.*Med. Sci. Sports Exerc.,* 37, 1381-6.

Hunt. S. A., Baker, D. W. & Chin, M. H. (2001). Guidelines for the evaluation and management of chronic heart failure in the adult.*J. Am. Coll. Cardiol.,* 38, 2101-2113.

I National Consensus on Cardiovascular Rehabilitation (1997). Arq. Bras. Cardiol. 69(4), 267-291.

Brazilian Institute of Geography and Statistics (IBGE) (2009). Studies and research - demographic and socioeconomic information. Rio de Janeiro (Sociodemographic and Health Indicators in Brazil - 2009, n. 25).

Irigoyen, M.C. et al. (2003). Physical exercise in diabetes mellitus associated with systemic arterial hypertension. *Revista Brasileira de Hipertensão,* 10(2),109- 17.

Jannig, P. R., Cardoso, A. C., Fleischmann, E., Werlang, C. C., Carvalho, T. (2009). Influence of the order of execution of resistance exercises on post-exercise hypotension in elderly hypertensive patients. *Rev. Bras. Med. Esporte,*15(5), 338-341.

Jones, H., George, K., Edwards, B., Atkinson, G. (2007). Is the magnitude of acute post-exercise hypotension mediated by exercise intensity or total work done? Eur. J. *Appl* Physiol.,102(1), 33-40.

Kaplan, N., Mendis, S., Poulter, N., Whitworth, J. (2003). World Health Organisation (WHO)/International Society of Hypertension (ISH) statement on management of hypertension.*J. Hypertens.*, 21, 1983-92.

Kelley, G., MacClellan, P. (1994). Antihypertensive effects of aerobic exercise: a brief metaanalytic review of randomised controlled trials. *Am. J. Hypertens.,* 7, 115-9.

Kenney, M. J., Seals, D. R. (1993). Postexercise hypotension. Key features, mechanisms, and clinical significance. *Hypertension,* 22, 653-64.

Krinskil, K., Elsangedy, H. M., Soares, I. A., Buzzachera, C. F., Campos, W., Silva, S. G. (2008). Acute cardiovascular effects of resistance exercise in hypertensive elderly women. *Acta Sci. Health Sci.* 30 (2), 107-112.

Kokkinos, P. F., Narayan, P., Fletcher, R. D., Tsagodopoulos. D., Papademetrious, V. (1997). Effects of aerobic training on exaggerated blood pressure response to exercise in African-Americans with severe hypertension treated with indapamide +/_ verapamil +/_ enalapril. *Am. J. Cardiol.*,79, 14246.

Laterza, M. C., Rondon, M. U. P. B., NEGRÃO, C. E. (2007). Antihypertensive effect of exercise. *Revista Brasileira de Hipertensão,* 14(2), 104-111.

Lee, L. L., Arthur A., Avis M. (2007) Evaluating a community-based walking intervention for hypertensive older people in Taiwan: a randomised controlled trial. *Prev Med.* 44(2), 160-6.

Lizardo, J. H. F., Simoes, H. G. (2005). Effects of different resistance exercise sessions on post-exercise hypotension. *Rev. Bras. Fisioterapia,* 9, 289-95.

MacDougall, J. D., Tuxen, D., Sale, D.G., Moroz, J. R., Sutton, J. R. (1985). Arterial blood pressure response to heavy resistance exercise. *J. Appl. Physiol.,* 58, 785-90.

MacDougall, J. D., Wenger, H. A., Green, H. J. (1991). Physiological testing of high performance athlete InTesting *strength and power* (2ª ed.) Human Kinetics, p. 39-40.

MacDonald, J., MacDougall, J., Hogben, C. (1999). The effects of exercise intensity on post exercise hypotension. J. Hum. *Hypertens.,* 13(8), 527-31.

Maher, C. G., Moseley, A. M., Sherrington, C., Elkins, M. R., Herbert, R. D. (2008). A description of the trials, reviews, and practice guidelines indexed in the pEDro database. *Phys. Ther.,* 88(9), 1068-77.

Matsudo, S. M. M. (2001). *Ageing & physical activity.* Londrina: Midiograf, p. 60-70.

Miranda, R.D., Perrotti, T. C., Bellinazzi, V. R., Nobrega, T. M., Criedoroglo, M. S., Toniolo Neto, J. (2002). Hypertension in the elderly: peculiarities in pathophysiology, diagnosis and treatment. *Rev. Bras. Hipertensão,* 9(3), 293-300.

Miranda, R. D., Perrotti, T. C. (2002). How to reduce blood pressure in the elderly? *Rev. Bras. Hipertensão*, 9,75-79.

Mokdad, A. H., Marks, J. S., Stroup, D. F., Geberding, J. L. (2004). Actual causes of death in the United States, 2000. JAMA,291(10), 1238-45.

Moraes, W. M., Souza, P. R. M., Pinheiro, M. H.N. P., Irigoyen, M. C., Meddeiros, A., Koike, M. K. (2012). Physical exercise programme based on minimum weekly frequency: effects on blood pressure and physical fitness in elderly hypertensive patients.

Negrão, C. E., Rondon, M. U. P. B., Kuniyosh, F. H. S., Lima, E. G. (2001). Aspects of physical training in the prevention of arterial hypertension. *Revista Hipertensão,* 4(3), 26-8. *Rev. Bras. Fisioter.* 16(2), 114-121.

Negrão, C. E., Rondon, M. U. P. B. (2001). Physical exercise, hypertension and baroreflex control of blood pressure *Rev. Bras. Hipertensão*, 8, 89-95.

Oigman, W., Neves, M. F. T. (2005). Isolated systolic arterial hypertension. InFrancischetti, E. A., Sanjuliani, A. F. (Org.). *Tópicos especiais em hipertensão arterial*(pp71-83). São Paulo: BBS Editora.

Oliveira, K. P. C., Vieira, E. L., Oliveira, J. D., Oliveira, K. R., Lopes, F. J. G., Azevedo L. F. (2010). Aerobic exercise in the treatment of hypertension

and quality of life of hypertensive patients in the Ipatinga Family Health Programme. Rev. Bras. Hipertensão,17(2), 78-86.

Oliveira, M. M., Damasceno, V. O., Lima, J. R. P., Galil, A. G. S., Santos, E. M. R., Novaes, J. S. (2011). Hypotensive Effect of Resistance Exercises Performed at Different Intensities in the Elderly. Rev Bras Cardiol. 24(6), 354-361.

O'Sullivan, S. E., Bell, C. (2000). The effects of exercise and training on human cardiovascular reflex control.J. Auton. Nerv. Syst., 81, 16-24.

Overton, J. M., Joyner, M. J., Tipton, C. M. (1988). Reductions in blood pressure after acute exercise by hypertensive rats. J. Appl. *Physiol.,* 64, 74852.

Park,Y-H., Song, M., Cho, B., Lim, J., Song, W., Kim, S. (2011). The effects of an integrated health education and exercise program in community- dwelling older adults with hypertension: A randomized controlled trial. Patient Education and Counseling, 8(1), 133-137.

Paschoal, M. A., Siqueira, J. P., Machado, R. V., Petrelluzzi, K. F. S., Gonçalves, N. V. O. (2004). Acute effects of low-intensity dynamic exercise on heart rate variability and blood pressure in normotensive and mild hypertensive individuals. Rev. Ciênc. Méd., 13(3), 22334.

Pescatello, L.S., Franklin, B.A., Fagard, R., Farquhar, W. B., Kelley, G. A., Ray, C. A. (2004). American College of Sports Medicine position stand. Exercise and hypertension.Med Sci Sports Exerc., 36, 533-53.

Poppel, M. N., Hooftman, W. E., Koes, B. W. (2004). An update of a systematic review of controlled clinical trials on the primary prevention of back pain at the workplace.Occup Med (Lond).,54(5), 345-52.

Proper, K. I., et al. (2003). The effectiveness of worksite physical activity programmes on physical activity, physical fitness, and health. Clin. J. Sport. Med., 13(2), 106-17.

Rebelo, F. P. V., Benetti, M., Lemos, L. S., Carvalho, T. (2001). Acute effect of aerobic exercise on blood pressure in controlled hypertensive patients submitted to different training volumes. *Revista Brasileira de Atividade Física e Saúde,* 6, 28-37.

Rêgo, A. R. O. N., Gomes, A. L. M., Veras, R. P., Drumond Jr., E. A., Alkimin, M. N. R., Dantas, H. M. E. (2012). Blood Pressure after a Supervised Physical Exercise Programme in Hypertensive Elderly Women. *Rev Bras Med Esporte,* 17(5), 300-304.

Robitaille, C., Dai ,S., Waters, C., Loukine, L., Bancej, C., Quach, S., , J., Campbell, N., Tu K., Reimer, K., Walker, R., Smith, M., Blais, C., Quan, H.

(2012).Diagnosed hypertension in Canada: incidence, prevalence and associated mortality. *CMAJ,* 184(1), E49-56.

Rondon, M. U.P. R., Brum, P. C. (2007). Physical exercise as a non-pharmacological treatment for hypertension. Rev. *Bras. Hipertens.,* 10, 134-7.

Rueckert, P. A., Slane, P. R., Lillis, D. L., Hanson, P. (1996). Haemodynamic patterns and duration of post-dynamic exercise hypotension in hypertensive humans. *Med. Sci. Sports Exerc.,* 28, 24-32.

Brazilian Society of Cardiology, Brazilian Society of Hypertension and Brazilian Society of Nephrology. V Brazilian Guidelines for Hypertension (2006).

Brazilian Society of Cardiology, Brazilian Society of Hypertension, Brazilian Society of Nephrology (SBC, SBH, SBN). V Brazilian hypertension guidelines (2007). *Arq. Bras. Cardiologia,* 89(3), 24-79.

Brazilian Society of Cardiology, Brazilian Society of Hypertension and Brazilian Society of Nephrology. VI Brazilian Hypertension Guideline (SBC, SBH, SBN). (2010). *Rev. Hipertensão*, São Paulo. 13(1), 6-66.

Shanhueza, S., Mascayano, M. (2006). Impacto del Ejercicio en el Adulto Mayor Hipertenso. *Revista HCUCh*, 17(2), 111-128.

Simão, R. (2004). *Physiology and Exercise Prescription for Special Groups*. São Paulo. Phorte Editora.

Souza, A. R. A., Costa, A., Nakamura, D., Mocheti, L. N., Stevanato Filho, P. R.,Ovando, L. A. (2007). A study on systemic arterial hypertension in the city of Campo Grande, MS.*Arquivos Brasileiros de Cardiologia,*88(4), 441-446.

Taylor-Tolbert, N. S., Dengel, D. R., Brown, M. D. et al. (2000). Ambulatory blood pressure after acute exercise in older men with essential hypertension. *Hypertension,* 13, 44-51.

Terra, D. F., Mota, M. R., Rabelo, H. T., Bezerra, L. M. A., Lima, R. M., Ribeiro, A. G., Vinhal, P. H., Dias, R. M. R., Silva, F. M., (2008). Reduction of Blood Pressure and Resting Double Product after Resistance Training in Elderly Hypertensive Women. *Arq Bras Cardiol*. 91(5), 299-305.

Topol, E. J. (2005). *Treatise on Cardiology* (2ª ed.). Rio de Janeiro. Editora Guanabara Koogan S.A.

Véras-Silva, A. S., Mattos, K. C., Gava, N. S., Brum, P. C., Negrão, C. E., Krieger, E. M. (1997). Low-intensity exercise training decreases cardiac output and hypertension in spontaneously hypertensive rats. *Am J Physiol: Heart Circ Physiol,*

273, H2627-H2631.

Verhagen, A. P., de Vet H. C., de Bie, R. A., Kessels, A. G., Boers, M., Bouter, L. M., et al. (1998).The Delphi list: a criteria list for quality assessment of

randomised clinical trials for conducting systematic reviews developed by Delphi consensus. J. Clin. Epidemiol.,51(12), 1235-41.

Verhagen, A. P., Karels, C., Bierna-Zeinstra, S. M., Feleus, A., Dahaghin, S., Burdorf, A., et al. (2007). Exercise proves effective in a systematic review of work-related complaints of the arm, neck and shoulder. J. Clin. Epidemiol., 60(2), 110-7.

Weinberger, M. B. (2007). Population aging: a global overview. In: Robinson, M.; Novelli, W.; Pearson, C.; Norris, L. (Ed.). *Global Health and Global Aging. San Francisco: Jossey-Bass Books,* Chap. 2. p. 15-30.

Whelton, S. P., Chin, A., Xin. X., He, J. (2002). Effect of aerobic exercise on blood pressure: a metanalysis of randomised, controlled trials. *An. Intern.* Med.,136, 493-503.

Williams, M. A., Haskell, W.L., Ades, P.A., Amsterdam, E. A., Bittner, V., Franklin BA, et al. (2007). Resistance exercise in individuals with and without cardiovascular disease. *Circulation,* 116, 572-584.

Willianson, J. W., McColl, R., Mathews, D. (2004). Changes in regional cerebral blood flow distribution during postexercise hypotension in humans. *J. Appl. Physiol.* 96, 719-24.

Wong, L. L. R., Carvalho, J.A. (2006). The rapid process of population ageing in Brazil. *Revista Bras. Est. Pop.*, 23(1), 5-26.

Yuvaraj, B. Y., Nagendra, G. M. R., Umakantha, A. G. (2010). Prevalence, Awareness, Treatment, and Control of Hypertension in Rural Areas of Davanagere. *Indian J. Community Med.* 35(1), 138-141.

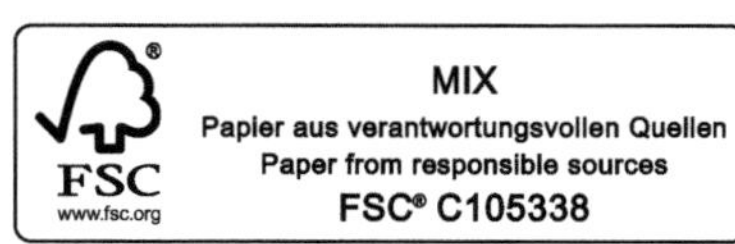

Printed by Books on Demand GmbH, Norderstedt / Germany